Diabetes: Learn About Type 1 and Type 2 Diabetes

Diabetics Handy Guide to Diabetes

By: Alex Klein

Notice To Readers

The information contained within this book serves to give a deeper understanding of Diabetes and its implications. The scope of Diabetes is vast and thus all information cannot be a universal information source for all diabetics. The best source of custom information for person 'x' will always be person 'x' doctor.

Table Of Contents

What is Diabetes and What Will It Mean for Me?

The diagnosis of diabetes can be confusing and cause a number of questions and complications. Diabetes can be controlled with proper diet and exercise, but unfortunately, it can be fatal if not treated properly. Therefore, it is crucial to understand this condition so you can care for yourself upon diagnosis of diabetes.

To put it simply, diabetes occurs when the body's blood glucose is not in balance, thus distressing the process of metabolism. Glucose is used by the body as a source of fuel. The body's cells need this fuel to carry out their processes and to keep the body moving. When the body can burn glucose, one can function properly rather than experiencing sheer exhaustion.

The body breaks down carbohydrates and the tract of the intestines discharges the glucose. The liver is in charge of grabbing the glucose and storing it for later use as glycogen. Some of the glucose circulates and enters in the blood where it will stay until it is needed.

Insulin is a hormone secreted by the pancreas. This function of this hormone is to carry the glucose. Circulating through the blood, the glucose and insulin bond together and the glucose is sent to cells in need. Glucose is permitted in the cells because the glucose likes the insulin.

When a person has diabetes, their body does one of two things. Either enough insulin is not produced for the body or the body's cells have created sensitivity to insulin which prevents it from binding with the glucose. Both of these situations cause the body's blood sugar levels to dangerously peak. One reaction, which is felt immediately by someone with diabetes, is exhaustion from not receiving adequate fuel.

What Implications Can Carbohydrates and Weight Have on this Diabetes Condition?

Although carbohydrates are fun to eat, we must keep in mind their implications. One risk factor associated with diabetes is obesity. When considering obesity, what matters is how one got to that point. What foods were eaten to gain that extra weight? Enjoying carbohydrates like bread products causes the levels of blood glucose to rise dramatically. It is important to keep in mind that the body turns carbohydrates into sugar. Continuing a high sugar and high carbohydrate eating regimen for an extended period of time may prevent your body's ability to make sufficient insulin to offset the consumption of excessive sugar. Down the road, this type of eating behavior can become a diabetes diagnosis and cause other problems.

Various body systems are also at risk by high blood sugar levels. For instance, damaged nerves resulting from high sugar levels are a common diabetes complication. The extremities of the fingers and toes often lose feeling because of nerve damage. Normal feeling in these areas would cause one to react if one burned their hands on the stove or stepped bare foot onto a sharp rock. Unfortunately, someone with nerve damage lacks this important feeling and may not feel the normal sting until the wound was very serious. The wound can also take an extended time to repair which is another complication of diabetes. Sometimes, these wounds can become even more dangerous when and if they lead to conditions like gangrene, which requires amputation.

The kidneys are another organ affected by diabetic complications. Often times, people with diabetes will need to urinate repeatedly. This is due to the natural mechanism of the body freeing itself of surplus sugars. The kidneys were not made to handle excessive sugars in the body.

Diabetes can wreak havoc on your body, especially during periods where the diabetes is not under control. Therefore, it is important that you understand what diabetes is, how to manage it, and how to keep away from serious complications.

Keeping a Watchful Eye on Glucose Levels

In review, the body utilizes the fuel resulting from carbohydrates processing into glucose. When your bloodstream has an excessive amount of glucose flowing throughout your bloodstream, this can lead to diabetes. A diagnosis of diabetes introduces the importance of managing your levels of glucose or your levels of blood sugar.

There are two types of diabetes which are called Type 1 Diabetes and Type 2 Diabetes. Type 1 is typically found in children and young adults. It used to be known as juvenile diabetes. This type does not generate insulin which is necessary in handling blood glucose levels. Type 2, on the other hand, is the most common form of this condition and the body simply does not manufacture sufficient amounts of insulin or the insulin is ignored by the cells.

Both types of diabetes sufferers need to monitor their glucose levels regularly each day. A diabetic with Type 1 needs to consider the fact that his or her body may not make any insulin to control the blood sugar level. A Type 2 diabetic needs to pay attention to the foods eaten as that may cause a spike in glucose levels. This spike may be above the amount of insulin secreted by the pancreas to be processed.

The number displayed on a glucose meter is your blood glucose number. It serves as an indicator of your body's ability to process the glucose and as a measure of your well-being as the day progresses. In the beginning, this process of checking your glucose levels will need to happen regularly, or until you become proficient in reaching your ideal blood sugar number.

What is the Purpose of Monitoring Your Blood Sugar Levels?

It is imperative to your health, for many reasons, to keep an eye on your glucose levels. Listed below are some of them:

• Avoid high glucose levels, or hyperglycemia
• Avoid low glucose levels, or hypoglycemia
• Successful management of diabetes and prevention of any complications
• Avoid heart disease

As shown by this aforementioned list, prevention is crucial. I hope you understand the importance of monitoring your glucose levels. Let's discuss further just how to do this.

How Do I Use This Glucose Reading Device?

The apparatus used to check blood sugar levels is called a glucose meter or a glucometer. The level is assessed at that moment from a minute blood sample. This information is useful during the before meal period and the period following a meal. By obtaining this information at these crucial times, you will know what amount of time is allowable from meal to meal, and if the foods you are consuming are the correct foods needed to control the blood glucose levels.

The market is flooded with various glucose meters so be sure to read the meter's instructions prior to using it. Blood is produced by a prick of the finger. The meter has a special spring-loaded needle and is preferred for its ease of use when pricking the finger. This assessment and finger stick process may feel unnatural in the beginning; however, the process will eventually become second nature to you. Blood taken from the finger's side is a wonderful suggestion for those with sensitive fingertips.

Please read the helpful steps below for using the glucose meter:

1. Make sure your hands are clean, washing with warm water and soap. The warm water will allow easier blood flow. Rub alcohol over the finger receiving the pricking.
2. Insert test strip into the meter which will power up the meter.
3. Remember the side of the finger is less sensitive. Stick your chosen finger, carefully, using the needle. Take your finger and milk it

gently allowing a blood drop to appear at the surface.

4. Hold the blood drop to the edge of the testing strip. Blood glucose levels will be ready within a few seconds.

5. Hold a new alcohol-applied cotton ball to your finger, using slight pressure. This will stop any new blood from coming to the surface and clean the finger.

The glucose reading on your device will give you a number. These numbers could be considered favorable or unfavorable depending upon the source. As a general rule, a favorable glucose level prior to a meal should read as low as 70 and as high as 99 mg/dl. Following a meal, it is possible to rise to approximately 180 mg/dl. (mg/dl. stands for milligrams per deciliter). Discuss with your health care professional a good range for your blood glucose levels. If the levels exceed the recommended levels, it should be brought to the attention of your health care professional. It might be an indicator that you are consuming an excessive amount of carbohydrates.

Glucose levels need to be monitored on a regular basis. By doing this, you will have the necessary information to manage your diabetes. This regular monitoring, along with a healthy nutrition and routine appointments with your physician, will help you manage your diabetes and minimize its complications and effects.

What Are A1C Numbers?

As mentioned previously, successful management of diabetes is gaining control over glucose levels. In fact, control over glucose levels is the most important objective. Blood glucose levels sustained at manageable levels minimizes resultant complications. This process happens over time in addition to finding stability from following your doctor's orders. Having careful consideration when doing so is important. This A1C number is a tool doctors utilize.

You may have heard A1C mentioned on a television commercial but you were unsure about how it associates with diabetes. The device for glucose readings (a.k.a. glucose meter) is routinely used to see where your blood glucose level is throughout the day. This number is crucial for treatment as it teaches you important factors in your diet. When are you consuming an excessive amount of carbohydrates and where is your diet deficient?

In the beginning of the journey with diabetes, you may feel uneasiness and confusion. You lack the understanding in the relationship between sugar and insulin and how critical it is to your health. Having Type 1 Diabetes means your body did not develop the normal mechanism to process the glucose. Because of this, you need to give your body the correct tool so it knows what direction to go. This process does not innately happen, otherwise.

An A1C number offers an expanded view of how you are managing your diabetes over a period of approximately three months. Perhaps this week it appeared as though you had an optimal handle over your diabetes, yet continued having symptoms. You can check your blood glucose levels whenever and receive a reading that signifies compliance, yet possibly that was not the situation during all the tests. It is at moments such as these where it is important to your health to get additional readings from your device.

A1C appears as HbA1C when written, and reads as "glycated hemoglobin A1C". Sugar is not alone when it circulates throughout your bloodstream. For instance, the blood is red in color from red blood cells. Hemoglobin is a protein that comes from the red blood cells. Hemoglobin attaches itself to iron present in the bloodstream.

In addition to binding to iron, hemoglobin is also able to attach itself to glucose. Because glucose is a sugar, it is also sticky. Over a period of time, unused glucose circulating throughout the bloodstream will attach itself to hemoglobin. The RBC's, or red blood cells, have the hemoglobin. Because RBC's remain alive for approximately three months prior to dying off, glucose can attach itself for quite a while.

What Does the A1C Number Determine?

These hemoglobin molecules in the RBC's are established and quantified by this A1C test. A percentage of attached, (or glycated) hemoglobin allows the physician to know what the median blood sugar levels are over that course of time. An average glucose reading would be approximately 150 mg/dl. This is scored by the A1C test as nearly seven percent. Eight percent or nine percent would indicate that your blood glucose level, at some time, was not under control. This A1C test is run approximately quarterly throughout the year.

These numbers give crucial information to your doctor. Your doctor can determine your blood glucose management with the previous information from the sugar monitoring records. This process assists you in managing your diabetes with control so your other body systems do not face danger.

Regular monitoring of your blood glucose levels is important, thus routinely use a glucose meter. In addition, it is vital to your health to schedule regular physician checkups for this A1C test. A greater knowledge concerning your diabetes will likely mean control of this condition and prevention of complications.

What is Hypoglycemia?

As we have thoroughly discussed, control of blood glucose levels is critical to diabetics. When glucose levels are under control, a diabetic will only need to alter their lifestyle minimally. However, when blood sugar is not well-managed and inconsistent blood glucose levels occur, a person with diabetes is in danger of complications such as hypoglycemia.

Let's Discuss Hypoglycemia

Even individuals who are absent of diabetes may feel weak following exercise or during periods of forgetting to eat. The term "hypoglycemia" may be used to describe them. While it is true that their blood glucose level may be dipping, hypoglycemia may not be the case. Individuals in good health may experience cases of hypoglycemia, which is low blood glucose. However, when a condition of diabetes is also thrown into the mix, hypoglycemia becomes a dangerous issue.

Just as we know blood glucose levels can rise to above normal levels, these levels also have the potential to fall dramatically below normal. This is also called, "insulin shock". This can adversely affect both Type 1 Diabetics and Type 2 Diabetics as they may both be reliant or non-reliant on insulin. Several factors can cause blood glucose levels to fall dangerously:

- You did not eat enough
- You did not remember to eat
- You over-exercised
- You consumed alcohol
- Your insulin was not under control

What Are Some Symptoms of Hypoglycemia?

When someone is suffering from hypoglycemia, the glucose found in the bloodstream is not in enough supply to deliver as fuel for the cells. Glycogen, defined as excess glucose stored over time in the liver, is used. Signs indicating hypoglycemia will start to appear. Some early indications include:

- Increased appetite
- Shakiness
- Sweating
- A fast heartbeat, or tachycardia

It is important to consume some source of glucose immediately, upon the first indication of hypoglycemia. Some options of glucose, or sugar, include glucose tablets, candy or perhaps a convenient on-the-go source of carbohydrate that is always with the diabetic sufferer. Having these sources available at all times is crucial to replenishing that necessary glucose. In most cases, these episodes occur often prior to bedtime or after awakening, thus storing some sources of sugar in a nightstand is smart.

The brain is one organ that needs glucose. As glucose levels dip, the brain does not function as optimally. Over time, dangerous low glucose levels can cause:
- Feeling faint
- Bewilderment
- Disorientation
- Becoming aggressive
- Diabetic coma

During this state of hypoglycemia, a diabetic might feel as though they lack energy to move about, and even if they could move, they would be confused. If a diabetic suffers from these symptoms, it is likely they require some glucose source immediately. They also need attention from a doctor right away.

To the person who has had diabetes for a long time; they may not recognize the signs of an episode of hypoglycemia. Feeling this way may be typical to them which could cause them to ignore the symptoms. On the other hand, it can also occur in the diabetic who was not taught the signs to look for during a hypoglycemic episode. It is for these aforementioned reasons that this information holds such importance.

If you or someone you know suffers from diabetes, gain all the information on the symptoms of hypoglycemia and how to treat hypoglycemia. If you have had diabetes for years, learning new information is still critical. You have power and can better manage your diabetes when you have knowledge.

What is Hyperglycemia?

A person can develop diabetes due to the abnormally high levels of glucose in their blood. This is termed hyperglycemia and is threatening to an individual who leaves it untreated.

Let's Discuss Hyperglycemia

Blood glucose levels have a tendency to be all over the place. When sugar levels elevate, it disrupts and causes issues in other areas in the body. In a nutshell, this is diabetes. Over the course of time, regular periods of high blood glucose can lead to diabetes; however, sudden surges in blood glucose can lead to more abrupt consequences.

You may ask yourself why blood glucose levels elevate. One probable answer can come from consuming foods that are wrong for you. An excessive amount of carbohydrates consumed at one meal sitting can overload your body with too much sugar. When the sugar load is too great, the insulin cannot bear the load.

An additional cause is the body's lack of insulin. Possibly, your body is not producing a sufficient amount of insulin. Another reason is that an individual that has been prescribed insulin (for the purposes of Type 1 diabetes) may be receiving too little insulin. The Type 2 diabetic may be experiencing resistance from the cells towards the insulin.

What Are Some Signs of Hyperglycemia?

There are three signs that typically indicate hyperglycemia known as the "3 P's"; polyphagia (increased hunger), polydipsia (increased thirst), and polyuria (increased urination.

It is natural for the body to rid itself of excess glucose taken in and the kidneys offer a route for the body to lose surplus glucose. To make this happen, one frequently needs to empty their bladders. The loss of water from frequent urination will also cause one to be thirsty regularly and when glucose is not used properly, constant hunger will occur.

Monitor your blood glucose level. Readings higher than normal, like 200 mg/dl need immediate attention to bring it down.

How Do I Treat Hyperglycemia?

Exercise is a phenomenal option for treating hyperglycemia. Use that surplus glucose! Rigorous physical activity will burn off glucose as fuel and lower your blood glucose levels to where they are normal.

One point to consider here: When insulin is lacking in the body, the glucose needed by the cells cannot be transported. The result can be ketoacidosis. This condition is when energy is produced by burning fat and ketones are released. An excessive amount of ketones are hazardous to one's health and the body will do its best to rid itself of them. Additionally, where fat is being used to produce energy, glucose is not being used, which causes blood glucose levels to rise.

How will you know if someone is experiencing ketoacidosis? Listed below are some typical signs:
1.   The breath smells fruity
2.   Difficulty breathing
3.   Nausea or vomiting

Attention from medical personnel is needed immediately. A diabetic coma or even death can result from ketoacidosis.

How Do I Avoid Hyperglycemia?

- Do regular monitoring checks on your blood sugar levels. The meter device is a great way to accomplish this.
- When your glucose is elevated, follow appropriate protocols to safely reduce your levels.
- Exercise (unless the urine shows presence of ketones)
- Inject some insulin

- Control your diet
- Lower the level of stress in your life

Remember, just as glucose levels can drop dramatically, your glucose levels can also spike uncontrollably. The resulting effects can be disastrous for your whole body. Having knowledge of what to look for and the treatment of high blood sugar (or hyperglycemia) will give you an edge to manage the outcome. Having vital information is crucial to the person who has diabetes.

Therapy with Insulin for the Type 1 Diabetic

The Type 1 Diabetic often does not produce enough natural insulin to manage the glucose circulating throughout the body's bloodstream. Various therapies are used to care for the person with diabetes. One common method is insulin therapy.

Let's Discuss Insulin

Insulin is a hormone that is naturally produced in the body. The pancreas secretes this hormone when the blood glucose levels indicate their need. When glucose or fuel is needed by the body, the pancreatic response is to secrete insulin. The cells need glucose transported to them. When the level of glucose exceeds the level of insulin, blood glucose levels can go higher than normal.

Type 1 Diabetics do not have the normal insulin producing capabilities. In fact, little or even no insulin is produced by the body. This causes a dangerous situation for the body to deal with elevated blood glucose levels. These dangerous effects include damage to eyes, damage to nerves, inadequate healing of wounds and damage to kidneys.

Medicinal insulin was acquired through many methods and many varieties of insulin exist today. In the beginning, animals provided insulin and the insulin was developed for human purposes. Unfortunately, the factor of rejection adversely affected the condition. Today, insulin is acquired by a process of creating human insulin through recombinant DNA. Having this source offers a lower probability of rejection.

What is Insulin Therapy?

Those individuals with Type 1 Diabetes depend on insulin therapy. The insulin is injected every day and occasionally more frequently than once per day to avoid blood glucose levels from above-normal elevations. Additionally, glucose needs to continue transporting fuel to cells. When an individual is insulin dependent, their blood glucose levels should be checked regularly each day. This monitoring ensures blood glucose levels are stable.

In addition to various insulin sources, various insulin types also need consideration:
- Standard or Regular
- Intermediate acting
- Long acting
- Rapid acting

Depending upon the blood glucose management plan, one or more of the above types of insulin may be prescribed by your doctor to manage your diabetes.

The insulin's time of onset is critical. It establishes the speed at which the insulin will drop the blood sugar level. The Rapid Acting Insulin begins dropping blood glucose levels in under fifteen minutes whereas Regular Onset Insulin could take nearly sixty minutes to drop blood glucose levels. Regular Onset Insulin is used in situations in which an individual's glucose levels are elevated, yet still out of the danger zone, such as following a meal. At times like those, lowering blood sugar levels rapidly is unnecessary.

The Long Acting and Intermediate Acting Insulin products would be useful for the diabetic individual who is experiencing good control of their diabetes with proper nutrition, exercise, and insulin. The person whose sugar levels are stable over long periods of time would be a great candidate for the aforementioned insulin therapy program.

Medically, there is some important residual information from trying insulin and succeeding or not succeeding. This is necessary when on an insulin therapy program. It takes careful consideration by your physician and yourself to check how you are progressing and alter your method of therapy when necessary. This process can take time to work at, so do not fret. Read and review the instructions from your doctor and be proactive with your diabetes.

Insulin Delivery Methods

Insulin, secreted by the pancreas to control glucose levels in the blood, is crucial to the body. When the body does not make insulin, the resulting condition is diabetes. In the past the only method for insulin delivery was via injection. However, other methods exist for diabetics today.

In regard to insulin, variables such as duration and peak times must be considered in deciding which delivery method is best for you. Insulin has a time when it is most efficient in dropping blood glucose. This is referred to as peak time. Duration is the amount of time the insulin will stay in your body and do its intended job, following the time the insulin was administered. Rapid acting insulin can act quickly; however, it might also last over the course of an additional one or two hours in the body. It is for these reasons that duration and peak times are vital when your doctor determines the insulin type and system of delivery.

Insulin Injection Method

Insulin via injection is the most common method. It entails a prescribed dose of insulin taken a certain amount of times per day and is injected with a needle or a syringe. The injection site is in the fat tissue as this type of tissue allows the insulin to absorb quickly into the body's bloodstream.

Your physician will go over proper protocols on self-injection. Remember, this process might go slowly in the beginning; however, it eventually will become second nature. Below are some additional reminders:

- Get organized with supplies first so that you have a moment to sit, get comfortable, and calm your nerves
- Make sure your hands are clean prior to touching the needle and insulin
- Use products that are sterile. Take an alcohol swab to run over the insulin bottle top. Use a new unopened syringe.
- Shake the insulin bottle prior to using it. The insulin can become apart from the solution when stored in the refrigerator. Draw up the number of units prescribed by your doctor.
- Ensure the site of injection is clean by utilizing an additional alcohol swab. Pinch and grab the skin with the index finger and thumb using one hand while the other hand does a 90 degree injection of the needle. Make sure the needle makes contact with the hub and the plunger is pushed down.
- Get a special container, called a "sharps container" to keep all used needles. These stored needles will need to be disposed of later.

The Insulin Pump

Persons with Type 1 Diabetes also have the insulin
pump delivery method, also prescribed by a doctor.
A little pump is connected to a catheter placed under
the skin, often the abdomen. Short-acting insulin is
delivered throughout the day. The ease of the insulin
pump gives a diabetic freedom in their life and daily
activities while insulin is administered.

However, a learning curve exists. A schedule needs
to be adhered to and numbers need to be put in.
These details can be discussed with your physician.
The catheter can be disconnected from the pump for
increased motion for activities such as showering,
jogging, and swimming. Remember, your medical
health team will assist you each step of the way until
you feel comfortable with the insulin pump method.

The Insulin Spray

This is a new method of insulin delivery. The insulin
spray is predominantly for Type 2 diabetics and
works similarly to an inhaler used by asthma patients.
Patients using this type of device need to have
adequate lung capacity to effectively bring insulin
into the system. Smokers would not be candidates for
the insulin spray.

Today, diabetics needing insulin do not necessarily
have one choice for insulin delivery. The syringe or

needle method no longer stands alone. Speak with your physician about the other methods available to manage your diabetes.

Drug Therapy for the Person with Type 2 Diabetes

Insulin therapy, for the Type 2 Diabetic, may not be necessary in all scenarios. Proper diet, medication, and a fitness routine can often control Type 2 Diabetes. You will learn below the various prescribed medications that control blood glucose levels in diabetics.

Upon the first diagnosis of diabetes, a change in lifestyle is a primary discussion topic by your doctor. Your risk factors today will be one of these primary discussions. These factors include poor nutrition, inactive lifestyle and obesity. As you begin making changes in diet and adopt a more active lifestyle, your physician may push the envelope by prescribing particular medications to get you where you need to be in a shorter amount of time.

Blood glucose levels still need to be monitored despite Type 2 Diabetics not taking insulin. Monitoring blood glucose gives useful information on the effects of their exercising and dieting efforts. Unfortunately, pricking of the finger is still necessary for management.

Medications

Diet, as previously discussed, is a large factor in managing diabetes. The effects of not eating food you should eat can be very damaging to the well-being of a diabetic. Eating non-compliant foods, such as a piece of cake or a cookie can cause your blood glucose levels to rise. This is due to the excess glucose circulating into the body's bloodstream.

Drugs that are Anti-Hyperglycemic

These medications are administered orally and can give great relief to the individual who dislike needles. The purpose is to drop your blood glucose levels via stimulation of the body's innate process of making insulin. One of these medications is Metformin, also called Glucophage. It lowers the liver's output of glucose manufacturing.

An additional job of this medication is to assist in making the cells more inviting to insulin which is important for the diabetic with insulin resistance. For individuals with stroke and heart attack risk, this medication has another benefit in reducing levels of blood cholesterol and blood pressure. This drug is particularly helpful to the diabetic struggling with excess weight.

Sulfonylurea is an additional class or type of drug that is beneficial in lowering blood glucose. Their function is raising the body's insulin manufacturing through natural stimulation. This is particularly useful to the diabetics that are suffering from limited insulin secretion and are not controlling their levels of blood glucose.

Another drug intended for diabetes management is Precose. Precose works in the tract of the intestines to lower the quantity of carbohydrates absorbed by the intestines. Once the process of breaking down carbohydrates is complete, glucose is transported through the intestinal walls where it circulates in the bloodstream until needed. When a reduced amount of glucose is available to the body's bloodstream, the quantity of insulin produced by the body can be managed.

Type 2 Diabetics that need more than just insulin to control their diabetes sometimes need an injectable drug that is a companion to insulin. If their blood glucose levels are not easily managed with only insulin, a companion drug such as Byetta and Symlin are used for more control.

Your physician may use only one medication, many medications, or even a combination medication to control your diabetes. The risk factors in your life, any additional diabetic complications, and whether you are managing your diabetes effectively or ineffectively with fitness and diet determines what medication scenario your doctor will prescribe. All of these treatment options should be a topic of discussion with your medical team professional.

Diabetic Foot Care

Diabetes is considered a metabolic condition which adversely affects the body in different areas. This is true even for successful treatment protocols. One area of the body rarely thought of by most people is the feet. When you have diabetes, proper foot care is paramount to the body's well-being and also to the body's health.

The Feet that Work Overtime

There is no doubt that your feet are putting in overtime as they work so hard. They support all of your body's weight. In addition, they put up with life's little dangers like being stepped on, toes being stubbed and even sharp objects cutting them. Despite the beating endured by our feet, they still keep on keeping on.

Sometimes the feet are affected by diabetes, yet it goes unnoticed. Remember, diabetics will need longer healing time for their wounds. Damage can occur to the foot's blood vessels and nerves in addition to the rest of the body. For example, one tiny cut on the sole of the foot may go unnoticed. That small cut could become a sore that did not heal and did not receive proper care. Eventually gangrene could set in and this would be terrible news to a person suffering from diabetes.

Giving Love to Those Feet

Let's make sure you know what to do so the above scenario does not happen to you. Your hardworking feet deserve special care. Follow these tips listed below to ensure healthy feet:

- Thoroughly study your feet on a daily basis. In the morning, take the time to look at your feet from all angles and in the spaces between toes. You are looking for spots that look suspicious or any wounds (even minor wounds). Even areas that might have produced irritation to the foot, and thus caused redness, need attention. Small irritations can turn into serious issues if they are not addressed.

- Wear cotton socks. Cotton wicks moisture away. Too much moisture provides an excellent atmosphere for bacterial growth which can lead to an infection. Even damp feet are prone to chafing, which causes irritation and sores over time.

- Wear comfortable shoes. Ensure some room in the socks and shoes you wear. If they are too restrictive, circulation can be cut off and eventually can give way to other issues. If the arches of your feet are problematic, consider gel supports. Gel supports are placed inside the shoe and offer improved comfort.

Do not wear shoes that fit improperly. One pair of shoes, or even two pairs, which offer a great fit, is crucial. You may want to seek out assistance in this process from a reputable shoe store.

- Seek immediate attention from medical professionals if/when you have foot issues. While self-diagnosis and treatment may be tempting for small complications like a foot blister, avoid this thinking. Perhaps you opened the blister and allowed it to drain or removed the skin layer over the blister. These dangerous treatment methods might start an infection of the foot. An open wound might occur which will be difficult to properly heal. The bottom line is to refer anything suspicious on your foot to the proper medical professional.

- Eat with sensibility. Managing your blood glucose levels aids in the health of your feet. Nerve damage prevention is so vital to foot health. Too often, injuries have progressed to a serious level because an individual did not know they stepped on a sharp object and the foot is cut. This aforementioned scenario, along with many others including nerve damage can be avoided by managing your diabetes with a sensible diet.

While everyone can benefit from good care of the feet, diabetics have even more to gain. Avoid serious issues in the future by following these above steps, today.

Diet for the Diabetic

Nutrition, fitness regimen, and medication are the treatment protocols for those with Type 2 Diabetes. Insulin is incorporated into the Type 1 Diabetes equation for managing blood glucose levels. For both of these cases, your physician may desire that you follow a diet specific to diabetes. This special diet should assist in stabilizing blood glucose levels.

Please note one "official" diet for diabetes does not exist. Rather, the American Diabetes Association set forth guidelines to aid in the management of diabetics blood glucose levels. This is regardless of taking or not taking insulin. Weight loss is also induced by this diet for diabetics dealing with excess weight.

Before you start any diet, it is important to discuss the plan with your doctor. The doctor plays an important role on your team for diabetes control, partnering beside you. The nutritional requirements specific to you will be influenced by various factors.
- The diabetes type you have
- Additional factors of risk are present (being overweight, disease of the heart, disease of the kidney, elevated blood pressure, elevated cholesterol, and so forth)
- Whether you do or do not need insulin
- Control of diabetes with drugs, or with nutrition and exercise alone
- Lifestyle that is active or non-active

So, let's begin with the typical meal that you consume. Divide the plate into three different sections of carbohydrates, protein, and fats.

Carbohydrates are used by the body to supply fuel following the breakdown of the food. Your meal needs a minimum percentage of 55 to 60% carbohydrates.

Any carbohydrate will not work. Eating foods that are minimal in calories and elevated in fiber is encouraged. Some great choices include beans, vegetables, whole grains, and fruit.

Ensure the foods are "whole grain" rather than processed white flour made to appear as a whole grain.

Protein is the body's building block. Every cells needs contact with this building block at one time or another. Lean meat, dried beans, lentils, fish, and peas are great choices. A maximum of 20 % of the meal should come from protein.

The body requires fats for many purposes. Fats that have the greatest benefit are mono-unsaturated and poly-unsaturated. Try using vegetable oil, olive oil, peanut oil, and canola oil when choosing oils. The body uses fatty acids that have Omega-3 to promote a healthy heart and improved immunity. Cold water fish are a wonderful source of Omega-3.

Approximately 25 to 30 % of the meal should come from this.

It is crucial that meals coordinate with the medication timing and injections of insulin to receive their most optimal use. Snacks are available for eating prior to bedtime or after you awaken to normalize blood glucose levels. A fitness program you can follow is helpful in reducing your blood glucose, and needs consideration in the insulin and eating equation. The individual with Type 2 Diabetes, particularly, needs to remember weight loss has the potential of bringing you a step closer to stopping any of the diabetes medications forever.

If you have diabetes and need to manage your blood glucose levels, a specific diet is mandatory. No single diet is referred to as a "diabetic diet". However, the aforementioned guidelines will assist you in the path that is best for you with direction from your physician. A nutritionist can also play key roles in this plan.